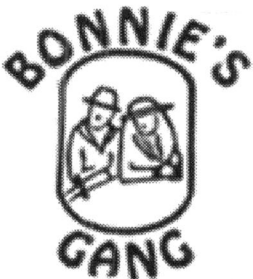

Bonnie's Gang Publishing is proud to present:

The third in a series of works for lovers.
Also by Jani:

The G-gasm Method

BlowPons ... Blowjob Coupons

Tonight's The Night

*... Your Ultimate Guide to
    Sexy, kinky
        things to do
            with your lover.*

Bonnie's Gang Publishing

Long Island, New York

Bonnie's Gang
PO Box 956
Melville, NY 11747

http://G-gasm.com
http://tonightsthenight.net
http://blowpons.com

Copyright 2006 Bonnie's Gang

All rights reserved
Including rights to reproduction
in whole or part in any form.

First Edition

Tonight's The Night is a registered trademark belonging to Bonnie's Gang.

ISBN: 0-9762090-5-5

Forward

Sex is the fuel that keeps love burning hot. Burn baby burn.

Use these coupons on complete strangers or give them to your lover, one that you have very strong feelings for already, nothing in between.

Pick a time and place where the two of you can spend some time looking through the ideas presented here. Some ideas you might giggle at, some you will toss out as "not for you," others you will pursue with pure lust. Enjoy them. Pick one out, and give it to your lover. Or, put the coupon in an "I Love You" card, and leave it by their morning coffee.

Great sex is beautiful -- two lovers creating their own music. Sometimes that music is soft and sweet, other times it is loud and rough. I like it rough.

How do you like it?

Enjoy!

Jani

Rub your fingers, against my opening,

By now, I'm sure to be wet. Don't penetrate yet ... make me suffer.

Bite and kiss ... lick my neck ... my breasts

While you rub yourself against me...

Grab the hair at the back of my neck ...

Force my head backwards ....

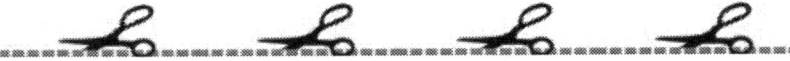

Tonight's The Night
... Sexy, Kinky Things to Do with Your Lover.

A Bedside Book.

To my wife Bonnie,

A wonderful lady,
with whom to share my life
and who loves me as I do her.
Not only is she the love of my life,
but also my best friend.

Thank you for everything.

Cock Worship

Tonight's The Night I please your cock. You know how indecisive I am. I have to use many different strategies to pleasure you.

I start with a hand job. I begin by gently placing my hand around your cock. I soon tighten my fingers to tease you and switch speeds to continue to make you want more. As you start humping and trying to ride my hand, I fall to my knees and take you in my mouth.

"I love your pulsing, leaking cock, the feeling of you being in my warm mouth."

My lips waste no time pleasing you. I slide you down my throat. My teeth toy with your shaft, lightly trailing up and down as I suck. My lips tighten around you, causing friction as I fuck you with my mouth. I can taste the precum, leaking out, coating my tongue. I lick the underside of your dick, forcing more of your love juices to ooze out - for my pleasure only.

As you begin panting and twitching, I know you are going to cum soon, so I stop. This does not mean it's the

Continued …

end. Instead, I straddle you to ride your cock. I want you to cum inside me, but not yet.

I slowly tease my cunt lips against the tip of your throbbing head. I moan out of pleasure as I feel your hard shaft stoke the fires of desire within me. I want you to enjoy the sensation for as long as you can.

My wetness slides down along your rock hard shaft, tight walls gripping you in a vice. My sweet nectar dribbles along your cock, as I ease it inside me. Your cock is throbbing as my cunt walls tighten and quiver. The smell of sweet sex fills the air, and I begin to rock, slowly at first as our bodies adjust to your cock inside me.

You fill me completely. Your cock is so thick and my hole is so tight that the smallest movement makes me cry out in the pleasure I feel, the desire I have to please you. I begin to rock faster until I am bucking against you, riding your cock like a wild cowgirl in a rodeo.

"Oh Baby, I love you!"

Our cries of desire fill the air, and as you thrust up inside me, I slam down on your cock. The throbbing grows more intense. I can feel it against my walls. My walls are clenching your cock as they quiver madly and I feel the pleasure flood my being.

I know that you are near orgasm, I scream out a throaty, "Yes! Baby you are the best!"

Continued …

I feel myself bursting from the intensity of it all. I feel a flood of pleasure. Your hot, white creaminess spurts up my pussy. My walls grip you tightly and I explode as my own orgasm bursts through my entire body. I continue to bounce on you as you thrust into me one last time.

... "Thank You, Darling."

A Night of Porn

Tonight's The Night we watch some porn. The movies are in the DVD player, we have quite a collection, enough for the whole night!

I lead you to the bedroom and stand there while you slowly, gently undress me. I undress you and pull back the sheets. Once you are in the bed, relaxing, I turn on the first movie.

The sound fills the room because I know you like it loud. As the movie starts, I curl up against you, as you watch the beautiful girls on the screen suck, and fuck. There are two horny women on screen, a beautiful redhead and a blonde. The two girls are rubbing one another as a sexy stud fluffs his cock in front of them.

I whimper and move closer to you, getting more excited than I thought I would. My hand slides to you and begins to pump your cock as the man on the screen is pumping his. Before you know it, I am simulating the girls on screen. I have a serious fetish for viewing porn ... I love the visual side of sex -- seeing it -- turns me on almost as much as doing it.

"Please let me suck your cock, I want to taste you."

Continued ...

The words leave my lips as I continue to stroke your cock, and slowly it gets rock hard in my hands. I follow the girls on the screen and pull your cock to my lips, greedily, and I suck it like a trained whore. My lips devour your cock as I suck you down my throat, bringing vibrations up and down your body. I suck your cock all the way into my mouth until I am swallowing you and there is not an inch left in the cool air.

I continue to suck you as your eyes watch the whores on the television until I can feel your cock twitching. I know what's going to happen. I know you're going to cum. That is when I pull your cock out and stroke you hard and fast with my hands.

"Cum for me ... Please cum I need your fucking cum" I growl out as I stroke.

I stick my tongue out and drink your cum as it shoots on my face. I smile with a twinkle in my eye and lick your love nectar from my face, curling up with you ... teasing your softening cock as we continue to watch these dirty movies all night long.

No Cumming

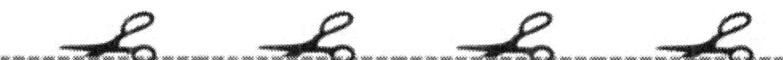

Tonight's The Night we kiss all night. I have not shaved today so you are able to feel that slight edge of stubble that I know you like so much.

My hands run through your hair as my lips meet yours. Soft kisses pressed to your lips -- my tongue slides out in search of yours. I move your body closer to mine. I hear soft sounds leave your lips.

I can feel your body heat rising as you press against me, as my hand moves around the outer curve of your blouse to touch your breast. I flick a thumb over your nipple, pressing in until I feel it popping out to press against my finger's persistent rubbing.

I kiss you for hours. I kiss you hard just as I would fuck you, but I will not fuck you, at least not tonight. Instead, I leave you horny. I make you want me, but no release.

My lips caress yours all night. They travel from your lips to your neck and back again. I nibble your bottom lip and suck on your tongue. My hands travel your body and feel the heat that our bodies make when we press together.

Continued ...

I kiss you until you are dripping wet and I can smell your sweet scent. Maybe if you are good I kiss your pussy. Soft sweeps of my tongue to clean up your wetness or maybe ... it just makes you wetter.

I move back up to your mouth again and kiss you softly.

"Remember, no cumming tonight!"

You look up at me and say, "Oh my god you mean you are going to leave me here like this!"

I groan in delight at the sound of your pleading but do not plead too much because all you get tonight are my kisses and nothing more.

One Free Flogging

Tonight's The Night you make me beg. Blindfolded, you lead me into the garage. You start by removing my top and letting my chest feel the cool air as your hands brush over my shoulders. Slide my skirt from my long, slender legs and leave it on the ground beneath me. Rip my bra from me; expose my body so that anyone passing by could see me. Leave on my panties. The thong I am wearing is nothing more than a small strap of lace. Maybe, if I get lucky, you will rip them off later. Your commanding voice tells me to remain still -- I do as demanded.

First, I think you are going to tie me up, but you do not. Instead, the first thing I feel is the soft yet commanding crack of your flogger against my skin. The leather strands are gentle against my back but I know that this is just the beginning. I ask for more.

I imagine your wrists twisting back and forth as the flogger smacks across my back, legs and ass with each stroke. I can feel the strokes getting harder with each flick of your wrist. My breath is quickening and I am getting excited. I can feel the wetness growing between my legs and I know you can smell my sweet scent.

Continued …

You continue for a while, moving the whip between my ass and thighs, and I can feel the heat rush to my ass cheeks and legs as they turn a delicious pink from the flogging. I wonder if you know that you are fulfilling one of my deepest and most humiliating fantasies. I have always wanted a serious ass spanking, and as painful and degrading as it is, I am enjoying every single moment.

The strokes get harder and my creamy flesh turns a crimson red. "Please Master, don't stop. Pleasure yourself with my flesh and your flogger," My words, filled with soft, broken breaths as pleasure fills me and I know you are pleased.

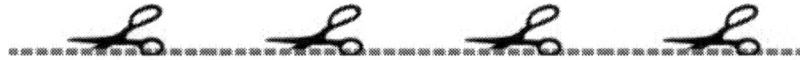

Man in Panties

Tonight's The Night we play with panties.

I bought some black lace woman's panties and I have them on under my clothes. I also purchased the matching bra for some added excitement because I want to turn you on.

I come to you and take your hand. I kiss it and slide it in my pants. I grin boyishly as I see your surprise.

"Is that lace?" you ask, and I nod. "I love a man in panties. They are so sexy on you."

You unbutton my slacks, pull them down, and see my panties rubbing against my hardening cock. My precum is oozing through the lace. You bend over to lick the cum through the mesh. I chuckle as you rip open my shirt to see the bra. My hands move to your ass and hike up your skirt, lifting you up to straddle me. This allows my panties to rub against your crotch. My hard cock is grinding against you from under the panties making you even wetter than before.

I rip your shirt off, letting our chests rub together and lay

Continued …

you on the couch. As I place you down, I remove your panties and rub against you a few seconds longer. You feel the tightness of my cock as the soft lace rubs your clit.

Once I know you cannot take anymore, I pull my cock from the panties, through the leg hole, but I leave them on and fuck you. I ram my cock into you. I thrust in and out repeatedly, listening to you cry out as you feel my cock and the lace against you. I fuck you until you cum.

I stand up, and you get on your knees in front of me. My little cumslut wants to suck me off. Your mouth goes to work on my cock. Up and down. Up and down. I feel my balls starting to let go. You pull your face off my cock, still jacking-me off. You lick my balls and then look at me. "Now cum in my mouth," You say.

You go back to sucking me. This time you are making love to my cock, not just sucking it, but also your hand is still stroking me gently. I feel a finger from your other hand work it's way up my ass. You know how to please a man.

"Yes ... now I'm going to ... I'm cumming...." I look down and see your mouth wide open, ready for the load of your life. Your finger still screwed up my virgin ass. I explode, you jack me off into your mouth and then you swallow. We lay down in bed. Our bodies touching and our hungry mouths contacting whatever skin is near. Thoroughly spent, we sleep in each other's arms.

One Body Sundae

Tonight's The Night we eat! We have one quart of French vanilla Haagen Dazs ice cream, a warmer, hot fudge, caramel, a can of whipped cream, some cherries, and some nuts.

I remove the robe I am wearing. You see I am naked and have been thinking about this all day. My hands glide down my flesh as I lie down and spread my legs on the floor.

I grab the ice cream. You watch me squirm as I cover my pussy in delicious vanilla. A big scoop is hiding my love spot from you. Next, I pour the hot fudge, my cool skin greeted by hot sticky chocolate as it drips over my thighs. The melting ice cream creates juicy sweet goodness.

My eyes drift over to you longingly as I reach for the caramel. I moan softly as the hot and cold desserts mix. I reach for the whip cream and draw pretty designs with the creamy topping on top of your dessert. I sprinkle the nuts on the whipped cream and add two cherries on top. The cherries remind me of the head of your cock -- red, plump, delicious and ready to eat.

Continued ...

I am covered, my pussy filled with your dessert. You come closer. I watch as you kneel down to eat your cuntalicious sundae, one lick at a time. Slowly you lap up dessert, as you are not one to rush a meal. Lick by lick, bit by bit, my luscious pussy comes into view. You keep licking until my lips part anxiously waiting for your tongue. Skillfully you slide your tongue into my hole. You suck on my clit, and slide your tongue back and forth like a dildo. You circle my clit with your tongue.

Soon, I'm crying out, "That feels so good ... aaahhh ... I'm cumming!"

"Would you like seconds ….."

"Yesssss!"

A Night of Bondage

Tonight's The Night you tie me up. Start by removing my clothes and guiding me onto your chair. I see the silk scarves you have laid out.

"Silk scarves and toys, I love that" I say softly, shivering with anticipation.

You tell me to close my eyes. You reach beside the bed, pulling the blindfold from the drawer. Quickly you tie the blindfold around my eyes. You bind my right wrist to the arm of the chair and then do the same to my left wrist. You tie both of my ankles to the legs of the chair. I am bound to perfection and spread open wide as I cannot hide from your gaze.

You begin softly kissing my foot, you move up to my calves and to my inner thighs. I let out a sigh of delight as your tongue slithers across my now wet pussy.

"Mmmm, oh yeah baby," I shout.

You move upwards, licking my belly button, working your way towards my breasts. You gently suck my hard nipples.

Continued ...

"Please, please, suck my nipples baby, God I love you sucking on my stiff nipples." I groan loudly, as you tug my hard breasts.

You slip your mouth upwards towards my waiting moist lips. You place your lips on mine and slide your warm tongue into my waiting mouth.

Suddenly, you stand and I hear you leave the room. I thrash wildly, to loosen the silk restraints, but to no avail. I sit quietly waiting for your return, my now drenched pussy pulsating with excitement.

After what seemed to be an eternity, I hear you reenter the room. I feel you getting closer to me. You get on your knees and kiss my wet pussy. You move up and place your lips on mine. The taste of my own pussy juice drives me wild.

"You taste incredible," I manage to say.

You slip your finger down to my slit and wet it with my slippery pussy juice, then you place your finger in my mouth ... I just about lose it just from that.

"Oh please, I want to suck you," I yell.

You take your cock out of your pants and slap me in the cheek with it. "I want to suck your cock, shove it down my throat and make me swallow your hot sweet cum like the whore I am."

Continued ...

I suck you incredibly well, and my mouth pleases your thick hard cock as you yell loudly. "Oh yeah." You shoot your cum into my mouth as I hungrily slurp up every last drop from the engorged tip of your swollen cock.

"That was incredible baby," you whisper.

You go back to the dresser drawer. You pull out my favorite vibrator ... soon it is buzzing my clit ...

"Oh, I'm cumming. I'm cumming right now!"

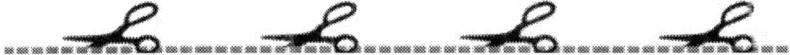

Nibbles

Tonight's The Night you wake me, by teasing me. Lightly run your hands over my breasts and toy with my nipples. You listen to my soft sounds, as I do not realize if I am awake yet or I am dreaming.

Breathe soft kisses down my stomach and let your hands trail down my sides. Trace your tongue over my belly button and down to my waiting pussy, blow on my clit as you spread my legs wider.

As I part my legs, you are able to slide one of your fingers past the folds of my outer lips and into the warmth of my waiting pussy. You feel me contract and begin to rhythmically hump your inserted finger.

I start grinding and thrusting before I even open my eyes. Soft peeps of joy leave my lips as you toy with me. I feel your tongue ease over my clit. Let it trace to my cunt but do not go inside. Make it last. Make me beg you to fuck me with your tongue.

Move your tongue around in circles. Tease me as it moves from left to right. Have it bump my clit. Nibble and suck on it, but do not let anything enter me.

Continued …

I open my eyes. My hands are grope to clench your hair. Now you really let me have it! You start licking faster and fuck me with your tongue. I scream in joy, as your tongue becomes relentless and your thumb finds that sweet spot that drives me wild.

I hump wildly against your face as my wails fill the room as I cum hard. Wave after wave crashes into me, as you continue to lick until I have nothing left and collapse into a satisfied heap, happy to doze off back to sleep.

Talk Dirty to Me

Tonight's The Night I want to hear that incredibly sexy voice of yours.

"What are you wearing handsome?" you ask playfully.

As I hear this, I immediately grin. "I'm wearing a suit and tie, my normal business attire. What are you wearing?"

"I am wearing very little. Actually I am lying in bed, wearing one of your neck ties."

"That's it?" I ask with a smile.

"Yep, that's it, just a tie. I woke up this morning after you left for work, and I was thinking of you so I decided to put something of yours on."

"What are you doing to my tie?"

"I'm rubbing it against my pussy, even though I'd rather be rubbing something else against it."

"What would you like to rub your pussy with?"

Continued …

"Your cock. I want to feel you inside me. I want you to fuck me. I want you to bend me over and take me from behind. Explore me. Use my mouth, my ass, and my cunt. I want you to cum in every hole and anywhere else you want. I want you to take me for your pleasure. Can you handle that?"

I feel my cock growing in my pants. My door is closed, but I can see everything happening outside the office. However, I know anyone could walk in at any minute.

"It sounds like a lot of fun, but I'm at work."

I grow harder as you start to whisper softly, "It makes me so wet to imagine your hard dick inside me. Touch your cock for me?"

"Someone could come in the office at any time. I m not sure that's a good idea."

"Just put your hand in your pants. It'll be okay. Come on, I'm rubbing my cunt for you and it is so wet."

My hand slides in my pants as I hear your sexy voice. My dick is incredibly hard.

"Are you rubbing?" You ask in your soft, silky tone of voice. "Are you touching, rubbing, playing with that huge thick, meaty cock of yours?"

"Yes I am. Tell me what you're thinking about."

"I'm thinking about you fucking me on the balcony. Continued …

Remember the other night when we were watching people walk by and you had your hand over my mouth so they wouldn't hear me. You had me from behind but then you turned me around and wrapped my legs around your waist. It was so hot. I love it when you fuck me."

I can hear your voice getting louder and I rub myself faster as I see someone approaching my office.

"Someone is coming. I might have to go." I say and find that I cannot stop as I hear your reply.

"I'm gonna cum." You purr out as you start to scream due to the orgasm shaking your body.

"Cum for me." You say softly.

Despite the person edging towards my door, my cock begins to stir and I cannot help myself. Thick white cream oozes from my cock in a blissful, quick orgasm thanks to your relentless teasing. As the door opens, I hang up the phone.

"Need anything from the deli?" a coworker shouts.

"No … I'm all good to go."

Sexy Dinner Date

Tonight's The Night we play at a restaurant. Slide your hand under the table and grab my cock. Massage it over my pants and remark about how hard it is getting. I do not want you to stop when they deliver us our food. Sit close to me and act as if you are not doing anything wrong.

Let me feed you while you toy with my zipper and slide your hand in my pants. Your expert fingers find my cock in no time.

Run your fingers along my shaft as you take a bite of your meal. I do all the feeding as you handle my cock. I groan softly, only loud enough for you to hear as you continue to play with my cock.

Start moving your hand slowly and gradually increasing the speed. Rub my balls as your nails trail my shaft. Make me adjust my seating position, so that your fingers can drive me wild. Talk dirty into my ear and make me that much hotter.

Stroke your hand up and down my cock and whisper to me how wet you are. Tell me you want to fuck me right here and now. Tell me you want to lick the cum from

Continued ...

your hands once I explode. As the waiter comes over, you order dessert in your most coy and friendly voice, while I fight to regain a normal attitude.

Watch me close my eyes as your fingers become more persistent and rub me harder as our waiter brings us our dessert. I thank him, trying to act as though nothing is happening under the table.

I hear your sweet yet evil laugh as you begin to lick the whipped cream with your finger as I explode. I cum coat your hand as you eat your sundae and offer me a bite. You end up smearing the sundae on my lips and kissing me. As you pull your hand from my pants, you bring it to your lips and lick your fingers as you did the whipped cream. We finish dessert, and head home to some more hot action.

An Anal Evening

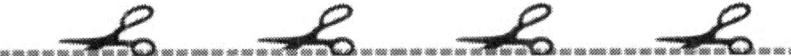

Tonight's The Night that you are a back-door man.

I have on that skirt that you love. You know the one I am talking about, the black silk mini-skirt that goes up to the mid-thigh. I bend over in front of you and show you I am not wearing any underwear.

You notice my creamy white thighs, the soft pink lips of my pussy and my rounded ass cheeks peeking out of my skirt invitingly.

You do not let me stand back up. With a firm hand you hold down my head, push me against the table, and leave my ass in the air. You spank me for being a tease and tell me what bad little girls get for toying with men.

"I'm going to fuck you in the ass, honey."

You unzip and pull down your pants. Rub the head of your cock against my ass cheeks to part them and let your cock play against my dark hole. I groan lightly, knowing how tight it is. Your precum is already oozing out to act as a lubricant.

"It's so big." I whimper as you push yourself in, "Ohh OHHH ...deeper... all the way ... aaahhhh..."

Continued ...

Rock against my ass and slowly feed me your cock. Pull my hips back towards you and begin thrusting in me slowly. Listen to my screams as your cock disappears up my tight ass and you begin spanking as you thrust.

Call me dirty names as you fuck my ass. Listen as my cries become louder and my tight hole forms to your thick cock. Fuck me harder now, do not stop, don't even consider stopping.

"Oooooh noooo don't do it stooop ooooh yes ooooooooh it's great, but you are too big - - but fuck me ooh yes fuck me ooooooh!"

Fuck me violently and make me scream for you. I know it makes you hotter when I scream. Feel my ass tightening around your cock, forcing you in and out. I can feel every little twitch inside my tight hole and I know when you are going to cum.

I stick my fingers in my pussy, and ask you, "Can you hear the squishy sounds my drooling cunt makes as my fingers slide in and out? I love those sounds, they make me so hot."

Spank me harder now. Fuck me harder now. Spray your hot cum inside me while you beat my ass. You know I want it as much as you.

"Yes, you are cumming. Cum hard for me. Don't hold anything back. Oh damn, you are so fucking good."
Continued ...

Your hips are working piston like as you pump your cock into my butt emptying yourself inside me. I can feel gobs of cum dripping from my hole. I turn around and give you a wink and a smile.

"I've never...felt anything like that...in my life... I love you Baby."

Master for a Night

Tonight's The Night that I am your Master.

As I prepare to go to work, I leave you with instructions for the day: Prepare for my arrival home from work.

That evening, I return home from a long stressful workday. You are waiting for me, kneeling on the floor in the living room. The only thing you are wearing is a black leather collar with a silver buckle around your neck. Your hands lowered to your thighs, your head raised proudly, your chin tilted up, and your eyes lowered gracefully in submission. I step into the room.

You greet me immediately by saying, "Welcome home Master."

As I smile and loosen the collar of my stuffy shirt, you immediately stand up and take my jacket. You loosen my tie. You unbutton my shirt, my chest exposed to the cool air.

I pull you into my arms and your pert tits rub against me. I let out a small chuckle at your exuberance, and I lift you. You manage to toss my jacket, shirt and tie, on the

Continued …

nearby couch and your long legs wrap around my waist. You can already feel how hard my dick is as it juts out against my pants. I carry you into the other room. You have already prepared the room to my specifications.

In the center of the room is a table, where I lay you down. There are leather restraints at both ends for your wrists and your ankles. I restrain you to the table. You try to yank your arms down, as they are above your head, but you cannot move them, and I laugh. As you tug at your bound ankles, your hips lift up and thrust into the air forcing your shaved sex to rise up closer to my face.

I lean down and lick along your clit, in a long slow tease. As I stand up straight again after licking your clit, I grab a feather. I run it along your ribs and neck. The feather teases around your breasts. I flick it over your nipple, first one, and then the other. The feather tickles and you squirm as much as you can, tugging on the restraints. I flick the feather down over your smooth tummy. The feather brushes along your glistening sex. I teasingly flick it against the folds brushing your clit repeatedly.

I reach for an ice cube from the bowl of ice you have prepared. I rub the ice against your pussy lips. I press the ice to your clit, rubbing it back and forth until it melts against your heat. By now your clit is numb, I lower my face to your cunt. I blow warm air on your clit, and you squirm.

Continued …

I dive my tongue between your folds and start licking furiously. The warmth of my tongue is such a different feeling from the numbing cold of the ice that you shiver against me. You are powerless, as you cannot move much. You must rely on me to please you, or torture you. I lick down to your hole and thrust my tongue inside you a few times, and my tongue flicks down along your crack as I rim your ass. I grab a vibrator from the tray.

I turn the vibrator on and thrust it deep into your cunt. By now, you are screaming in pleasure. My tongue is working against the crack of your ass, and it slips inside your tight little hole -- into the little dark star. I continue to rim you as I thrust the vibrator deeper into your wet hole. I lick the drippings of cunt nectar from your hole as it dribbles down your ass crack.

You yank against the restraints and beg me to let you out, but I do not. Instead, I zero in on your clit and lick you like mad. The vibrator is still thrusting deeply, in and out as it buzzes. I continue to lick, putting pressure on your spot, the spot that makes you cum. You scream and beg to cum as I lick and I pause, as though I am contemplating letting you cum. Finally I say you can cum, and you explode on my tongue, your honey spurting onto the slick vibrator as I continue to pump it in and out.

I lick you as you ride the waves of your orgasm, and continue to pump the vibrator as deep as it will go. You are spent. I stand up and pull the vibrator out of you. I

Continued …

turn it off and put it to your lips and you suck your juices from it. I put the vibrator back on the tray and release you from the restraints. Your legs are like jelly so I carry you into the bedroom where you lay against my chest.

As I nestle your body against mine you whisper a soft, "Thank you Master, you are the best."

Snowball

Tonight's The Night we have a snowball fight. I don't mean the kind people throw around outside on those cold winter days. I'm talking about cum swapping.

We have returned home after having a few drinks together at the bar. We are talking and laughing. I tell you that I feel a Popsicle growing between my legs.

You kneel down to get a better view; you just have to lick it. You lick it like a lollipop. You love the feel of my cock in your mouth; it makes you feel like a slutty little whore. You grab my cock and push it into your mouth as far as you can. You choke a little but you continue to suck on it. I start squealing with pleasure and a little bit of white, creamy stuff spurts into your mouth.

With your hand, you grab the base of my penis and squeeze gently, yet firmly, thereby not letting me explode. My dick is throbbing. A stream of cum is oozing from my swollen head. You lick it up, but you are careful to not swallow it.

You stand up, and grab the back of my neck with your hands and pull my lips to yours. Your tongue penetrates my lips, as you force the love juices into my mouth. We

Continued ...

kiss for what seems to be an eternity, swapping the cum back and forth between our mouths.

You get back on your knees to a now very engorged, red throbbing cock. You stick the head into your soft mouth. With your hands, slippery from your saliva, you stroke my cock up and down. Within seconds, I am exploding into your mouth.

"Oh, my God, I fucking love swallowing it! Oh my God," you keep whispering, eyes half-closed from pleasure, long pink tongue licking your sticky lips. "I love eating fuckin' cum! That was so fuckin' hot,"as a mixture of cum and saliva dribbles down the side of your mouth.

I kneel down. Hungrily I grab your neck and pull your lips to mine. We kiss and kiss and kiss ...

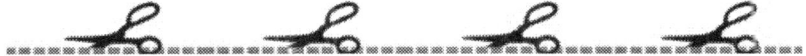

My New Cock Jewelry

"Bend over!" I command.

You ask me why and I tell you to just do it. You comply. You hike up your cute little skirt, and snap your thong. I tell you to take it off and you do. You hear me unzipping my pants, you try to turn, and look, but I push your head back.

"Don't Look!" I yell.

You are more than curious by now. I pull my cock free from my briefs. My cock springs from my tighty whities, and I rub the tip against you. You instantly feel the sensation and you gasp. I have been hiding it from you.

"What is that?" You squeal loudly, and your body wiggles back against it.

The round metal piece hits your clit and you groan low and loud. You rub against it, and I let out a blissful whimper as well. You do not care what it is. It feels so good. My cock is so hard, as I slide it back and forth against your slit. By now, you are already begging for more. You want me to slam it inside you, but I do not. I like teasing you. I like making you wait.

Continued …

Your wetness coats my new cock ring. I begin to rub harder against your nub. You squirm back against me, closer. My hands move around and move up your stomach beneath your top. You are not wearing a bra. I squeeze your firm, supple breasts. I pinch the nipples, as my cock rolls against you. I find your hole and rub the head around it.

I slam my cock inside you and the ring rubs against your clit. You are like a marshmallow now, soft and squishy. I am squeezing your breasts, massaging them, and rubbing the nipples as I thrust my cock inside you. I fuck you deeper, in and out, and your screams continue to echo through the room.

I pull out of you and let go of your breasts. You whimper in protest, but turn around to look. Your eyes widen as you see the cock ring and you drop to your knees. You begin to suck my cock. It slides in your mouth and against the metal. I close my eyes and thrust into your mouth. I ride your face; precum oozes into your mouth, which you swallow greedily.

I continue to pump your mouth, as you suck me like a trained whore. Your one hand is rubbing up and down my cock as your mouth sucks, licks, and nibbles softly along the head and under the shaft. Your free hand massages my balls, and the spot beneath my balls.

My cum is stirring within my balls as the need to explode fills my body. I continue to pump my hips as I fuck your face. Your continuous stroking of my balls and the shaft

Continued …

finally, make me detonate. I groan loudly as I explode in your mouth. The ring makes my orgasm more intense as you tug lightly on it with your teeth.

Thick gobs of creamy white cum shoot out of my cock -- over your tongue, splashing onto your cheeks. You hold my cock slightly away from your face, so that I can get the creamy jet right on your tongue. You gulp and swallow quickly, enjoying the warm thick taste. Plenty of love juices spatter on your cheeks -- a few drops on your forehead and some had escaped your lips and dribbled down your chin.

"I cannot wait for tomorrow night," I whisper.

Exhibitionist

Tonight's The Night I watch you with your best friend. You know the one I like, the leggy blonde with the big tits, Rebecca. You kneel in front of her and slowly slide her skirt down over her hips. Pull it off. Remove her panties with your teeth, and softly blow on her sex.

I am in the other room with the television on; perform for me. I am videoing you with the digital camera, which is transmitting a picture to the TV and Rebecca, does not know I am watching. I sit in my comfortable chair, leaning back, with my hands in my pants.

Bury your tongue in her hole. Thrust in and out so she can ride your face. I hear her moans of pleasure and you articulating at how good she tastes. Rub her clit and stroke it with your fingertip. Make her gasp and ask for more. Lay her down on the bed and spread her thighs.

Rub her puckered little asshole, and then when she is nearly cumming, move away from her cunt. Pull her skirt up above her head. Yank it off, and then have her help you remove your own clothes.

Once naked, you rub your tits against her cunt. Your nipples are hard, as they rub against her wet pussy lips.

Continued …

Move up her body and grind your hips into hers, then turn yourself around and kneel above her face.

Sixty-nine her. Make her eat your pussy as you eat hers. Bury your tongues in each other's cunt hole. Rub each other's puckered little asshole, and stroke each other's clit. Move in unison, as I pump my cock, my very hard cock.

Cum in each other's mouth as I spurt my white cream in the other room. Scream as you cum, knowing I am pleased at your display, and when she leaves, come in the room with me.

Kiss me, rub your tits in my cum, "Girl ... you are something else."

Your Sweet Little Slave Girl

Tonight's The Night I come into the room and kneel at your feet. I am wearing a covering of silk, and a leather collar but nothing else. The silk covers my body, but only enough so that I am not naked.

As I kneel down, my hands go to my thighs and my eyes lower. My thighs' part and you can see my shaven pussy is glistening in wetness at the idea of serving you. My voice is soft like spun silk as I ask, "How can I serve you Master?"

As I wait for your response, I do not look up. I feel you kick my legs apart and I whimper softly as they spread wider for you. My love hole is now open and waiting for your command.

I sigh as I feel the air hitting my spread open mound; the waft tickles my smooth, baby soft skin. You do not move. I am tempted to look up, but do not dare. I feel your boot scrape against my pussy. It presses against my clit and scrapes to open my lips even wider.

I untie your boot and slip it off. "Ride it bitch," you say with a frown and a scowl.

Continued …

At your command, my hips begin to rock against your foot. Soon I am coating your foot with my wetness. You shove your foot against my cunt and your toes' slide into me. You start fucking me with your foot. Your foot is slamming into me and soon I am crying out in pleasure.

"Harder whore" you growl at me as your foot slams into me.

I can smell the scent of sex as you rape me with your foot. My hips are humping and grinding. I keep moving faster and harder. My body is moving closer to cumming and I cannot stand it anymore.

"Please Master, please let me cum!"

You just laugh and kick up with your foot while it's in my cunt that causes me to lose my balance and fall off. You shake your head, laugh in my face, and only say one more thing, "Clean me off slut."

I start by cleaning off your foot - I lick your toes to make sure that there is no pussy juice left on them. As I look up, I see that you are rock hard and I beg pleadingly to see to your other needs. You tell me to remain where I am; you pull your cock out of your pants. You stroke it inches from my lips.

"Stick it in your mouth. Bitch," you command. Your cock begins to twitch.

Continued …

Your scorching hot cock twitched hard and a large spurt of pungent cum shot from deep within your balls. I swallow frantically, trying to keep up with the huge load that you keep firing into my mouth. I can't take it all in my mouth and you cum all over my face.

Then you make me lick my face clean like a dog using my fingers to get the hot steamy cum into my hungry little mouth. Then I lick your cock clean, only then am I finished.

"Thank you, Master," I say with ecstatic sincerity.

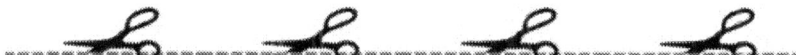

Dr. StrangeLove

Tonight's The Night I examine you.

Disrobe, and put on this small gown. Lie down on the table.

I spread your legs for you to make sure that I can see everything I need. I look at you adoringly for a moment before moving to your side.

I tell you I need to do a breast exam to ensure that your breasts are free of lumps. My hands move around your breasts, squeezing and pinching your soft white skin. You close your eyes and pretend not to notice me until I flick a nipple. I just smile politely and remind you it is part of the exam.

I sit on a stool and get between your legs. I run some cold gel along your cunt and rub it in until you are slick and smooth. You keep your eyes closed. You do not ask why, you just nod and a small smile appears on your lips. I start by pressing a finger inside you, as is procedure. My finger moves inside you, working in your cunt until it is much slicker then it was. You sigh softly and seem almost disappointed when I remove my finger. I replace my finger with a metal speculum (vibrator). It slides easily into you and I move it side to side, in and out.

Continued …

My finger rubs against your clit, as I tease the speculum around your opening, and then stroke it more vigorously in and out. "Everything seems normal so far. I just need to check a few more things. I need a larger speculum, so if you feel more pressure everything is fine. Just keep your eyes closed and I will be done before you know it."

I make sure you cannot hear me, as I move closer to you. My now hard cock is poking out of my shorts. I press my cock against your slick pussy. I press into you slowly and press down on your abdomen.

"That's good. Everything is going fine."

As I continue to push into your cunt, you gladly accept my cock. I feel your hips move up and I mutter that you need to sit still. My hand rests on your abdomen holding you down as I fuck you harder. My strokes are long and slow. Soon you began to groan and that changes everything. I become bolder and more excited. I fuck you faster and harder as you fight to move against my hand.

I do not let you move. I do not let you do anything but as I continue to pound in you, I can feel your cunt spasm and it forces me to cum. Your body tries to rock against mine as we both slip into orgasm. I slowly remove my cock and zip up my pants.

I sit back down on the stool and wipe you up. Once you open your eyes, you find an empty room and a bill on the table waiting for you.

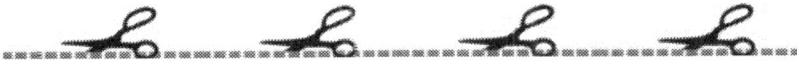

Lap Dancing

Tonight's The Night you dance for me. Exotic dancers get me really excited and hot. I want you to be my slut.

Put on some "bump and grind" music.

I take a sip of my drink and I tell you I'm ready for the show.

You start by standing in front of me, and slowly swaying your hips. Tease me with that sexual grind that only a true slut possesses. Once you have my attention, run your hands through your hair and down your beautiful body. Cup your breasts and turn from me. Rip your shirt off and let it fall to the floor. Remove your bra as you dance for me. Turn around with your hands covering your tits and make it obvious that as you grind you are playing with them for me.

Move your hands and glide them down your stomach towards your crotch. I want to hear you whimper as you remove your pants slowly and run your hands over your satin covered pussy. Rub your fingers into the material as you fall to your knees and spread yourself open. Pull your panties to one side and rock against your hand to

Continued …

the beat of the music. Let your whimpers of joy join the music as you fuck yourself for my amusement.

Look at my hard cock that continues to grow as I watch you roll over so that you can crawl to me. Slide your body up mine until you are straddling me, rock against my dick to the beat of the music. I grab your hips and rock you faster. Clothing separates us but still I will be able to feel your tight little hole teasing me. You whisper in my ear, as I feel the wetness from your panties against my jeans, "I love you sweetie."

The song ends; your hips slow -- your body stops moving...

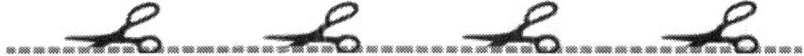

Threesome

Tonight's The Night you invite your friend to join us.

I come home and you are having a beer with your best friend Tim, that cute guy with the nice ass. As I move into the room, you pull me into your lap. I blush, and am slightly embarrassed. Your friend just laughs. You begin to rock my hips against yours in a slow grind and I turn to whisper in your ear that we have company. By now, my face is scarlet. You just grin and tell me he doesn't mind, and when I look at him, he wiggles his eyebrows at me to show he really does not care and actually seems to be interested in the action.

You stick your hand up my skirt and I squeal. I am so shy and I try to wiggle away but you hold me against you. I am constantly looking at your friend, and I can see his hand is resting against his groin. As I try to move away, you hit my sensitive spot and I begin to whimper. I ride against your hand and forget we are not alone in the room.

I do not even realize it, but the next thing I know my clothes are off and I am straddling your lap. Your cock is hard, steaming hot, and it is teasing my opening. Your fingers are sliding up and down my wet slit, never going into my hole, but moving up and down teasing me.
Continued …

I lean down to kiss you as I feel a nibble on the back of my neck. I gasp as your friend has come up behind me. He nuzzles and kisses my shoulders while his hands wander to my breasts and cup them, gently rubbing my nipples with his fingertips. I instantly look at you for approval. You just give me a horny little smile and slam me down on your cock. This is electrifying.

I can feel your friends hard on pressing against my ass. I am nervous at first, but I lean back a little bit and start to get into it. He is kissing my neck and toying with my nipples. He rolls them between his fingertips pinching them, squeezing them, and tweaking them as I arch my back and bounce on your cock. The movement of our rocking forces me back against Tim's cock and it slides up my tight asshole.

I thrust on your cock in my cunt and rock back on Tim's dick up my ass. Soon you are bouncing me between your bodies and I am screaming in my pleasure. I want you to both cum inside me, filling me with your hot, white, jizz.

"Fuck me like the whore I am, use my body for your amusement," I yell.

You continue to slam your cock into my pussy and Tim pumps away at my ass. You both begin to orgasm; your bodies shudder. My whole body fills with blissful pleasure. I can feel you both cumming inside me as my walls clench both cocks, holding them deep within my openings. I collapse against you, shot and spent. I turn around, and Tim is gone.

Switching Roles: My First Anal Experience

Tonight's The Night you bend me over and shove your strap-on dildo up my ass. Wow, I can't believe I said that.

I know that you have never cross-dressed as a man so I will help you look the part. We pick out some manly clothes. You are not the stuffy, up tight, businessman kind of person so the clothes are casual.

You wear a long sleeved designer shirt, with a jogging suit over it. On your head is a bandana. Your hair is up in a bun so it looks short, like a guy's hairdo. You sit with your thighs spread wide, as if you were a man. You are wearing boxers, but I can already see the outline of the strap-on dildo pressed against the fabric.

It makes me hard to see you like this. I want you to take control. Your lowered voice excites me. You stand, kiss me, grab my dick and pull me towards you. You keep your hand on my shaft as you guide me down the stairs into the bedroom. You pull me to your lap and call me your little sissy boy. I can feel the dildo press against my ass. I nod and tell you that I am anything you want me to be.

Continued ...

You push me to the floor and laugh. You stand up and remove the jacket of your jogging suit. As you remove your long sleeve shirt, I see you have a wife beater on beneath it.

You yank me up and bend me over your chair. You pull down my pants and spank my ass. Your dildo slides through the opening of the jogging pants. The head of the dildo cock presses against my asshole. You are nice and squeeze some lube against my virgin ass.

You press the cock into my ass. Slowly I become used to it. I moan and cry as it hurts, but then you press into my prostate and I nearly cum. You begin to rock, the tip teasing in and out of my ass slowly. You hand reaches around and fondles my balls and cock. I am really getting into this, and in no time, I am slamming my hips back against your cock.

The cock is so slick and it slides in all the way. It does not hurt anymore, and actually, I like the fullness. My cock is twitching and you are grunting. The manly grunts turn me on. I fuck back against the dildo and when I think I cannot hold on any longer you tell me I can cum. I grab my cock and after only a few strokes, I explode in orgasmic bliss as you continue to ram your cock up my ass, and rub my balls as I stroke the shaft.

I collapse into the chair. You pull out of me, your bitch boy, forever.

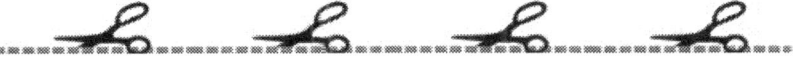

Mutual Masturbation

Tonight's The Night I watch you, while you watch me. We masturbate together.

You lie at one end of the couch and I lie at the opposite end so that we are facing one another. Rub yourself, especially your thighs ... I know how sensitive they are. Unbutton your pants, and slowly reach in and start to play with your cute little pussy. I do the same.

You take off your panties and throw them to me. I watch you suck your juices from your fingers and I sniff the scent of your moist panties. The sounds of your whimpers are driving me crazy.

You spread your legs so that I have a good view and my legs are open so you can see my cock. Start by tracing the outline of your pussy for me. I trail my hands over my cock for you in return. Perform for me as I stroke my cock for you.

My hand glides down my shaft and I clench my cock as I begin to stroke it for you. My other hand massages my balls. I watch as you stroke your pussy. You slide a finger inside your wet hole and let your cunt envelope that finger with your wetness. You add another finger and another because that is how big my cock is in your tight little hole.
Continued ...

Rub your clit and fuck yourself faster. Rub it fast and hard, as my tongue would be stroking it if I were to lick you. Beg me to stroke my cock and watch me as I do as told. I stroke harder and faster, my hips moving upward with each thrust of my hand. I start to groan as I listen to you cry in pleasure.

"Fuck, you sound good," is all I can manage to say.

I can see you are about to cum. Your hips are moving wildly on the couch, your juices running over your tight hole. It's driving me mad just to look at you. My own cock is more than ready to cum.

"Stop," you command. "Aren't you going to squirt your cum in my little panties?" you giggle.

As you stop I grab your hand, the one that has been in your cunt this whole time and I lick it. It's sweet with your juices and it makes me want more so I pull you up and onto my cock.

It only takes a few deep, pounding thrusts before you explode on my cock and as your walls tighten, I am ready to explode.

"Oh, Darling fuck me HARDER!" You cry, your firm little ass quivering wildly. "I'm cumming all over your big cock!"

Continued ...

You move off me and wrap you panties around my throbbing cock. You only have to stroke it a few times before I start gushing. My hot love juices cover your tiny little panties.

"Please, I GOTTA taste your big hot sticky load," you beg.

You get on your knees in front of me, and lick your semen-covered panties. With your fingers furiously rubbing your clit, the taste and aroma of our love juices mingled on your panties, you explode in a violent, almost scary powerful orgasm.

We collapse in a puddle of post orgasmic bliss.

Oily Massage

Tonight's The Night I give you a full body rub. I bought a set of body oils with all the essential slippery stuff needed to relax your tense muscles.

I remove your shirt. Your body is so sexy, and I cannot help running my fingertips over you. You remove your pants, and I give you a towel to wrap around your waist. You lay down on the padded table I have set up, with your face and stomach down into the padding. I stand to the side and open one of the bottles of oil. I drizzle the oil along your back. It is cool to the touch. It hits your hot skin, and you gasp, "Oh Honey that feel's so good."

I run my hands over the oil, and begin to knead my fingertips into the smooth skin. You are tense. I rub my hands over your shoulders, your shoulder blades, and down lower toward the curve of your back. I massage the oil into your flesh. I rub in a kneading circular motion I stroke my fingertips over your back. I am working out all the kinks in your muscles and soon you have a dreamy look on your face.

"Is there any other area where you feel tense?" I ask.

"Just keep going ... you're doing a great job."

Continued ...

I rub down your butt and your legs. All the stiffness in your joints, the tightness in your muscles seems to fade away. I pour more oil on your thighs. I finish massaging your backside -- you are so loose you are nearly floating on air. I ask you to roll over.

You roll over, and I can see your cock is hard, and is sticking up against the towel. I pour oil onto your chest and start rubbing it in. I flick and play with your nipples; this makes your cock undulate beneath the towel. Your muscles flex against my unrelenting hands. I move down your stomach, oiling it up as I go. Your stomach quivers as I run over the smooth, sensitive stomach skin. I dip beneath the towel and accidentally knock it off.

"Sorry about that," I say with an apologetic oops, as I looked down to see your cock fully hard and upright just inches from my hands and face.

I oil up your cock and wrap my hand around the shaft. Immediately, I start stroking it slowly up and down. I massage each oil-covered ball, squeezing them lightly. I then slide my hand back up along your cock. I am pumping furiously now and your body is writhing in ecstasy. You are fucking my hand as I give you an oily massage.

The surface of your cock is slick, creating more friction, and it does not take long before you are grabbing at me, and groaning in pleasure.

Continued …

"Ooohh ... Baby, that feel's sooooo good."

You thrust your hips in and out until you cum all over my hand. I milk the cum from you and smile. I clean you.

You are totally relaxed ...

Let's Not Get Caught

Tonight's The Night we go out in public and try something new. It does not matter where, but I think the mall would work fine. I want you to wear a skirt and hold my hand as we wander around.

"I have to go to the bathroom," I say to you. You nod and let go of my hand. I pull your hand back and smile as I whisper, "I want you to come with me."

You grin, seeming shocked for a moment and take my hand back, following me towards the bathroom. Together we enter the bathroom and proceed to the furthest stall in the back. With the door closed behind us, you begin to rub my cock through my jeans.

"So, Honey," you laugh, "What shall I do with you?"

"You can do whatever you want," I reply as I feel my cock push against my jeans.

You unzip my pants and stroke my cock. I just grin and do not move for a moment. I close my eyes as you stroke. It's an enjoyable feeling to have your hand on my cock.

Continued …

"Mmmm, what a nice hard fat dick you have for me today," you say.

I press you against the stall and hike up your skirt. Your hands hold onto the top of the door as you sink down on my cock. Your long legs wrap around my waist as I thrust into you.

Your cunt is so tight and my cock so thick that you get the urge to scream though the voices right outside the thin door would know what you were doing. I put my hand over your mouth and begin to fuck you harder. I fuck you quick, fast and hard. This fuck is dirty. The appeal of being caught makes it that much more interesting.

My free hand begins rubbing your clit. My hand presses into your little nub until your body is shuddering and bucking wildly against me. Your orgasm pounds through you. My cock begins to twitch from the tightening of your slick hole and my own orgasm rocks through me. Thick creamy juices shoot into you while you hold the door and try to keep your mouth shut.

Slowly I let you down from the door, easing my rocking and kissing your lips. I pull up my pants as you straighten your skirt and let you out of the bathroom as all the people stare and wonder but only we know the truth.

We are not caught ... this time.

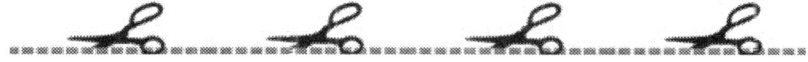

That New Vibrator

Tonight's The Night we play with a new vibrator. I bought you a present today. I know you have never had one, so I thought it would be interesting to control the buzz as it comes to life against your hot juicy pussy.

The idea came to me, that nothing is better than the element of surprise. I think I will wait to show you when you are sleeping.

That night, my hand slides under the covers with the new vibrator in tow. I rub it against your pussy lips, and you are slutty enough to open your legs when you feel the object because you think it is my cock. I continue to rub you, with your eyes closed, you whimper for me, rocking your hips lightly and spreading your legs wider.

Once I turn the dildo on, you react oddly until you feel the vibrations. It causes you to jump and your eyes shoot open. I waste no time and place the toy on your sweet spot, right against your clit. I stroke the vibrator in circles teasing your clit and listening to your sounds of delight.

Your body begins to shudder and you cry out that you want to cum, that you need to cum and you are going to cum. As you are saying that, I thrust the vibrator into
Continued …

your cunt and fuck you with it. I fuck you wildly. I watch you twitch and sigh loudly as you explode all over your new toy. Your orgasm is unlike anything that has occurred to you and the sensation something very new.

Your body calms. I remove the vibrator and put it to your lips so you can remove the juices and I can watch you eat your new toy.

You fall back asleep almost immediately ... exhausted, worn-out and happy.

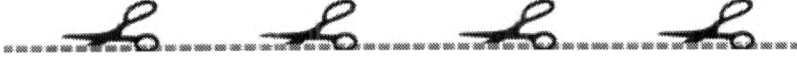

Golden Shower

Tonight's The Night you teach me a lesson. I have been bad. What are you going to do about it? Are you going to make me see the error of my ways or are you going to continue to let me be a bitch?

You need to humiliate me. Show me how little I am, how worthless I am without you. Tell me every flaw I have and laugh at me for them. Make me sorry I ever dared to upset you. Piss on me.

Pull me to my knees in the corner of the shower and turn off the stream of water. Smack me, if I protest. Tell me you are sick of my shit and you are not playing games anymore. Pull out your cock and smack me with it.

Ask me to apologize and shake your head when I laugh. Tonight is your turn to laugh. You start smiling as your hot golden piss squirts from your cock and splatters and drenches my body.

You watch as I try to get away from the strong steady stream, but there is nowhere to hide from the warm liquid. Trapped, I am unable to get away from it. The hot urine is shooting at me. It hits my breasts, my cunt, my hair, and everything. I curl into the corner but your cock continues to shoot at me.
Continued …

As the stream stops, I look up to see you masturbating and the next thing that hits me, mixing with your urine, is your cum. Equally as hot, though this is white and sticky, it lands all over my flesh.

You finish. You laugh as you look at me, covered in urine and cum. You call out before you leave the room.

"Clean yourself up and make sure you behave next time." You pause to laugh before adding. "I wouldn't want that to happen to you again."

"Think we could do this again sometime?" I ask.

Golden Boy nods, "Um ... sure." You shake your head as you turn to leave and shut the door behind you.

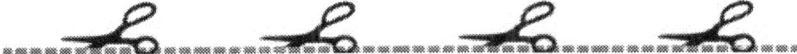

Working Girl

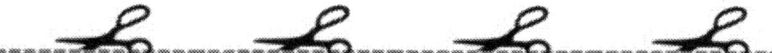

Tonight's The Night we have to work. I love that we work together because being your secretary does have its advantages. My favorite moments are when you call me into your office and tell me to take notes.

I like it when you put an anal plug in my ass and make me sit on it while taking notes. The vibration in my ass is so intense. Eventually it makes me cum during the note taking session. You just stand there and smile, but that's a different story.

Tonight is different. I come in; you lock the door behind me and tell me to sit on your desk. You have me spread my legs and hike up my skirt before putting the note pad in my hand.

You unzip your pants and press your cock against my wet pussy lips. You begin reciting the notes as your cock slams into me. You love a dirty game. You want to see if I will be able to stay on task while you try to distract me.

Your cock pounds harder and faster into me. Your words become quieter, more broken through your moans and grunts. I fight to keep up with the task but my writing is

Continued …

hard to read. I am thrusting and more concerned with your cock than any form of dictation that you want me to do right now.

"Oh yes fuck me hard, make me cum with you" I said as my orgasm began to rush through my body.

You stop as I begin to scream and you ask for my pad. You bend me over the desk and you spit on my ass before you slide your thick cock inside it. You push past the dark star and into the tight warmth of my ass. I SCREAM!

"Oh my fucking God!" I squealed. "This feels so different -- so good. I never felt like this before. So tingly. Big time. Big fucking time!"

You pull at my hips thrusting me back on your cock as my screams fill the room. You spank my ass as you fuck it and tell me to rub my clit. The pleasure is overwhelming. My ass filled, my clit buzzing from my fingers -- I still must take notes. I fight to stay on task but it is a losing battle. Soon all I am thinking about is my pleasure.

You stop and look to the pad and see that I have stopped writing and you shake your head. You have me sit back on the desk again and spread my legs. You begin stroking your cock and grunting as it is already so close to orgasm that it only takes a few quick strokes before you are cumming on my cunt.

Continued ...

I just love a pussy covered in cum. To me nothing is sexier than a huge load of cum shot outside of a pussy! I rub the love juices into my hole and then lick my fingers clean.

You make me wear your cum all day because I was a bad girl and couldn't take your notes right.

Ho! Ho! Ho!

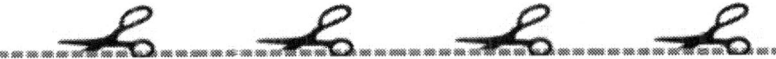

Tonight's The Night we visit Santa. I have always heard that Santa brings toys to good little boys and girls, but what about those of us that are not so good.

I want to sit on your lap Santa and convince you that I deserve just as much as those good little girls. I can be good too and I will do anything to prove that fact.

I come to see Santa just before he retires to bed. I ask to see the inside of Santa's bedroom.

You tell me that my behavior disappoints you. You received the list of naughty and nice and I was naughty. I would not get any toys this year.

"Please Santa. I need new toys. Mine are all worn out." I whimper and press myself against you as you tell me that I will receive nothing.

You frown and say, "You cannot sway me with your slutty ways girl! Naughty bitches do not get any presents."

I growl softly and fall to my knees, digging your cock out of your suit. I lick it like a candy cane and suck it like a trained whore that I am. My mouth moves up and down your shaft.
Continued …

My lips tighten as they fuck you and I pump harder as I feel you lean back and loudly exhale.

"Suck my cock like the slutty whore that you are," Santa orders. "Suck it you little tramp!" he grunts, thrusting his hips towards the back of my throat.

I suck you until you are about to cum, then straddle you on Santa's throne, my pink moist pussy lips are eager for action.

I ride you like a cowgirl begging and pleading for new toys. I promise to fuck your elves if you want me to and to be your slave girl on Christmas. Fuck the cookies. I will give you snatch, ass, and anything else you want.

"Just give me toys..." I begin pounding harder and faster, fucking Santa wildly, screaming out in pleasure and grabbing at your suit, shoving you in and out of my tight, wet hole. "Fuck me Santa! Make me your bitch! Make me work for those presents!"

Apparently, my tight cunt and dirty tongue are winning you over. When I lean down and suck on your ear you let out a scream and I feel your cum shoot inside me in hot long streams of pleasure. I thrust harder riding out your orgasm and mine until you push me off.

"See you Christmas Eve," you grunt pulling up your baggy red pants.

I'm Horny

Tonight's The Night ... I'm horny.

I was cleaning today and found some of your magazines. They were all of beautiful women naked. I have been reading them for hours and toying with my clit as I wait for you to get home.

With a few minutes left before you arrive home, I turn on one of your x-rated videos and slip a finger inside me just to tease myself.

As you come through the door, you can hear the television and my sounds of delight as I play with myself. You walk in to see the magazines scattered around me on the bed and my cunt spread wide with my fingers inside it. You notice the movie for a moment, but you have the real thing waiting for you, so you take off your clothes.

You hop onto the bed and shove my hand away. You sit on my face, feed me your cock, and shove your head down into my cunt sixty-nine style. Your tongue begins to lick ferociously as my lips suck you in and swallow your whole cock.

Continued …

You eat me with force. Your tongue presses hard against me and I return each lick with a lick of my own. My teeth tease your cock as you nibble my clit. I start to scream and hump against your face, pushing my head up in an effort to swallow more of your cock, even though I have it all in my mouth.

You feel as you are about to cum, you pull away from me and bend me over. You sink your cock into my tight hole and pound into me. While watching the girl on the DVD fuck two men, you ram me from behind doggie style. Your cock pounds into me, raping me harder with every stroke. I am screaming and bucking back against you. My juices are covering you and melding with your own pre-cum.

You grab my hair and start to groan. I know you are going to cum. I feel my own orgasm approach and scream as we both hit that destination at the same time.
.
You go faster. I grunt. You go harder. I moan. You tell me you want me to cum. Cum now for me, baby. I give in. I scream my cunt contracts rapidly. Oh, god yes, I am thinking. Yes. Yes. Yes. You kiss my forehead. I know you are close. You whisper, I'm gonna cum, baby, I'm gonna cum, now... One long last thrust and you collapse atop me. Panting. You kiss me. I snuggle into you. Hold me. You hold me. Your heartbeat and breathing are like a lullaby. I could fall asleep right now.

Continued …

"I love you Darling," I whisper. My body still shaking, we lay down.

We lay there like that for several minutes before I get up and stand by the bed. I lift my leg over your chest and rub my pussy onto your nipples spreading the love juices all over you.

"Again?"

Voyeur Time

Tonight's The Night we watch the neighbors. I noticed that our neighbors like to fuck with the window open and I want you to watch them with me. I want to sit on your lap and sit astride you while we watch.

We watch as the man presses the woman up against the window. It is so dirty that we are watching them and do not even know their names. He is spanking her and she is crying. She must have been a bad girl. He is rubbing her tears with his enormous cock. You start getting hard and I rock against your dick as we watch what happens next.

She takes him in her mouth and begins to suck him. He pulls out his cock every so often because he likes to beat her with it. This does not last long though because soon he bends her over. His cock slides into her ass and even though we are across the street, I swear I can hear her screams.

He does not wait. He pounds into her. He is rough and violent. It almost looks as if she is bleeding though I cannot be sure. My eyes lock on the scene. I know you can smell my wetness as I rock against you, feeling your hardness next to my ass.

Continued …

I gasp as he pulls his cock out and cums all over her. He scoops up the cum and feeds it to her out of the palm of his hand and a short sigh escapes my lips at the thought of you doing that to me.

He cleans his cock with her hair. He shoves his cock into her mouth. He chokes her with it. I watch as she fights against him and he eventually lets her go, tossing her to the floor.

The lights go out in their apartment. You grind against me.

Now it is our turn ...

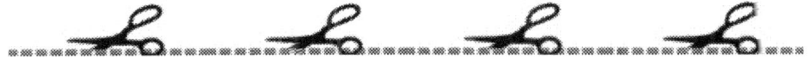

How Many Licks?

Tonight's The Night we play a new game. The name of the game is how many licks does it take. I want to know.

I start at your neck and give you a few licks. I check your reaction before I move to your ear. I remind you that once I am below your belly button I need you to count for me. You need to keep track of the licks I made from that point on.

I lick your neck and move to your ears. From your ears, I lick along your lips to your neck and I move down to your collarbone.

I move to your breasts and kiss along each one. I flick and tease each nipple. I nibble and lick them in alternate strokes until you are writhing and twisting under my skilled tongue.

I move down your body and lick down your stomach. I travel down until I am between your thighs. I listen as you keep track and I lick your cunt in a long slow stroke, paying extra special attention to your clit. You gasp out in pleasure as I repeat this process and slide my tongue into you repeatedly

Continued …

My tongue alternates from slow to fast but it is always persistent and soon you are rocking against my face. I shove my tongue into you. This only counts as one lick because I do not remove my tongue. I just continue to fuck you with it. You scream and grind down hard on my face; your juices cover my tongue and lips.

"My God!" you cry out. "You're makin' me cum so good! Here it is! I'm cumin'! Eat me! Swallow me!" As my tongue slows to a stop, you gasp for air and tell me that I made it in one hundred and ten licks. I laugh and exclaim that it will take more than that to clean up your love juices and my tongue goes back to licking you clean.

Fisting

Tonight's The Night we try fisting. Your fist is big, it might hurt a little but once in, I know it will feel good.

You lube up your hand and play with my pussy. Rub it gently and flick my clit to loosen me up. Watch me as I spread my legs and you slide a finger into me. Rub the finger inside me and start to fuck me with it. Fuck me slowly at first and add another finger into the mix.

I start to wiggle and struggle against you, but you add a third finger. My cunt is getting much tighter now as you add more fingers. Spit on my cunt and add a fourth finger.

"Put all of your hand in me," I gasp.

I feel myself getting full, but I want it all. Your fingers are working inside my cunt but it is so tight. The lube with my wetness make things so slick, you push your thumb inside me and now your whole hand is up my pussy.

Your hand curling inside me to form a fist, pumping in and out of me forces my muscles to contract. I scream and hump against your hand in a forceful orgasm.

Continued …

"I can't believe my whole hand is in your cunt," you say with a look of bewilderment on your face.

The violent orgasm wracks through my body. I push and rock against your fist, fucking myself harder and making my orgasm last longer.

"Oooohhhh, that is really good, isn't it gooooood, fuck, fuck me, harder. Oh god I'm cumming, I'm cumming, Oooohhhh fuck, don't stop."

As I finish cumming, you uncurl your fingers, remove them one by one, and then lick them off for your sweet little treat.

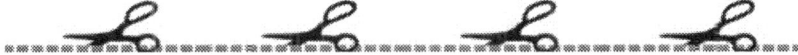

Wine and Dine Me

Tonight's The Night I dress up in my sexiest outfit. I am wearing a sleek, black dress with a plunging neckline that shows off my firm breasts. The slit of the gown goes up my long legs, and almost to my hip. My hair is elegantly pinned on top of my head, and I am wearing high heels with straps that wrap around my ankles and up my legs.

I walk into the dining room and I see you waiting at the table for me. You have on your best suit, and an erotic smile, just for me. I sit down next to you and you pop open a bottle of wine. It's a rare vintage, my favorite. You set the open bottle down on the table in front of you and pat your knee invitingly.

I move around the table and sit on your lap. You pour a little bit of wine on the top of my breasts and lick it off greedily. Your free hand is already moving my dress to the side. I run my fingers through your hair, as you lean down to suck each nipple.

Your plate filled with fine foods you love to eat; Filet Mignon with béarnaise sauce, whipped potatoes with gravy, asparagus and strawberry cheesecake for dessert sits in front of you. We take turns feeding each other steak, savoring each bite.
Continued ...

By now, I am sitting in your lap straddling you. I arch my back as you lick my tits, and focus on my erect nipples. My whimpers of pleasure fill the room. You are enjoying yourself, and you pull my dress down even more. Now I only have on my pantyhose, thong and shoes. You pull the pantyhose and thong down around my ankles, and pull me back down so I am straddling you again.

I feed you the asparagus, and we finish the steak. You pour more wine down the front of me, and this time it dribbles all the way down my body. You lick all the way up and down, drinking greedily from me.

We finish the main course. Dessert is next. You pick me up and lay me on the table. You smear cheesecake down my body from my tits almost down to my snatch. You smear some cake on my pussy lips, and a little piece on my clit. You begin your race down my body as you feast on the cheesecake.

I wiggle and beg you to fuck me. You lick along my breasts, on my nipples, down my stomach, past my belly button, over my abdomen, and along my pussy. You dive your face into my folds and lick the cheesecake off my clit. We finish the cheesecake. You pick me up and carry me off to the shower to wash me and....

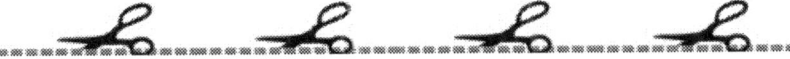

French Maid

Tonight's The Night you dress in a French Maid's uniform. You have the standard black dress on with a white apron, a white maid's hat, black stockings and black shoes with heels. I smile and nod as you dust around the room. You ask me if I need anything.

I am sitting in my chair, in the den, curled up with a book. I tell you I would like a cool beverage. You run off to fetch the drink for me. As you move toward me, you fall and the drink crashes to the ground. You look apologetic as I frown at you.

You get a dustpan and clean up the glass, "I'm sorry sir," you say with regret.

I force you to kneel before me, and you wobble down to your knees. I shove you on your back.

I move close to whisper in your ear, "This is your first lesson Darling. No orgasms without my permission. In addition, you will really have to beg before I let a slut like you have any pleasure; certainly not before you give me some."

Continued …

You begin to cry, and I call you a worthless sissy of a maid. This just makes you cry harder. Quickly you sit up, sobbing at my feet, babbling incoherently about obeying me and how you would be happy to eat my cock, to please me.

I tell you that you were a very bad girl. You just nod knowing you have disappointed me. I unzip my pants, and lower them to my ankles. You reach up, grab my briefs and pull them down ...

A Sexy Cyber Fucking

Tonight's The Night to log on to my computer. I love cybering with you. I know what your special name is and I approach you. Our conversation reads something like this:

Hotgurl4u22: Hey stud, I hear you have many girls hitting on you.

Stud121992: I am irresistible...so...tell me a little about you...

You always did get right to the point. Perhaps that why I enjoyed all the time I spent with you.

Hotgurl4u22: I'm 22 from Hawaii and of course, I am a female. How about you?

Stud211992: What a coincidence I am in Hawaii, too. I am 25 years old and I am a male.

Hotgurl4u22: That's really cool and stuff...so do you wanna fuck? (Leave it to me to get straight to the point.)

Stud211992: Sure. I grab you and pull you close to me. I can already feel my cock throbbing from your wetness.

Continued …

You are so incredibly attractive. I run my hands through your hair. What color is your hair?

Hotgurl4u22: Brown. It's long, in thick waves. I have 38 C tits, and I am 5'4. I weight 119 lbs. I also have green eyes. How about you?

Ok so this was a slight exaggeration, but this is how we always play and I know your cock is already hard from playing this little game with me.

Stud211992: I am 6'0 exactly. I weigh about 200 lbs. I bench press a lot, and have firm muscles, blonde hair, and blue eyes.

Again, an exaggeration, but the description still makes me hot, so I finger my hole with my free hand. I start to some sounds knowing you can hear me as our doors are open, and we are only a few rooms apart.

Hotgurl4u22: You sound so sexy. I want to jump on your lap, pounce you and rip your clothes off. I want your body so badly, your hot beefy body.

Stud211992: You're getting me hot -- I want to bend you over my desk, and show you how a real man fucks. I'll show you who's the boss.

(Oh, so you want an office scene. I smirk and continue to finger fuck myself as you use your typical "let me show you how a real man fucks" line.)

Continued ...

I know by now you can hear my whimpers and I imagine you are stroking your cock as you wait for my message.

Hotgurl4u22: I need a real man. I need a real cock... I want you to fuck me...I want to slam my hips down on your cock and bounce wildly.

Stud211992: Pens, papers, pencils, and paper clips will fly everywhere as we fuck. Moving wildly inside you and groaning low, "your cunt is so tight." I plunge in and out of you deeply, forcing your walls to accept the cock within you.

I am really getting into it now. I close my eyes and I am moaning loudly. Just as I am typing my response, you log out. I curse the servers, and the entire computer system. I know that they are all against me. I am in the moment and why else would you leave.

I reluctantly remove my hand from my cunt. My mood is about to turn sour, but just then you enter the room. You are naked. You heard my whimpers and got so horny chat was not enough.

You scoop me up in your arms, and carry me off to your desk …

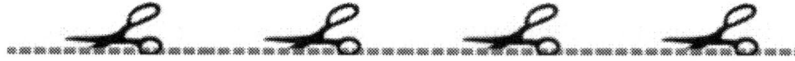

My Porno Queen

Tonight's The Night you are my movie star. I am the director and you, my porno queen. You are a good girl that has gone bad.

With my cell phone, I captured a digital of you masturbating on the bed. You writhe against the silk sheets, and whimper loudly as you hit all the sweet spots. You thrust your hips upward off the bed as you plunge a dildo inside your snatch. I catch you sucking your love juices from the dildo.

Just before your orgasm, as your eyes glaze over, you scream out my name unintentionally. As you cum, I zero in on your hot pussy, your glistening shaved snatch, and then move the camera to your face to catch your reaction to the explosion.

You are a little embarrassed, but we watch the digital together, and we both agree that you could b a porn star.

"I want you to fuck one of your girlfriends. Let me video the action. Start by getting in the 69 position; play with her asshole. Rim her, and use toys on her. You can use a double-sided dildo and fuck one another with it. Ride against each other. As you shove the dildo up your pussy, your snatch rubs against hers. Then, lick her clit

Continued …

until she cums on your face, and let her fuck you with a vibrator until you explode. It will be awesome, we'll have the scenes, and we will be able to watch them whenever we want."

"I want you to suck my friend's cock. Devour it as if it was mine. Suck it deep into your mouth, and let it hit the back of your throat. Slide your mouth up and down his shaft as you toy his ass with your finger. Fuck your finger into his ass and massage his prostate. Suck on his balls and then fondle them with your free hand."

"I want you to roll his balls around with one hand, and pump your fingers in and out of his ass with the other. Use your teeth to tease gently against his shaft. Suck it into your mouth and when he cums I want you to move back. He is going to stroke his cock as you wait, and then when he cums it spurts all over your face and breasts."

"Oh Baby, that sounds so hot," you say to me almost drooling at the thought, "when can we start?"

"All potential actresses have to have a personal try out with me first."

"Oooh yeah," you whisper.

Sex in the Shower

Tonight's The Night we shower together.

I open the door and hope it does not creak. It does not. I move across the bathroom floor and slip into the shower behind you. I wrap my arms around you and grab your cock. I stroke it as you yelp in surprise.

You turn around and pin me up against the wall. The hot, steamy water hits our bodies. You rub soap all over me. I kiss you with hunger and longing. You have only been gone long enough to take a shower, yet I miss you.

You lift me up and wrap my legs around your waist and your cock is pressing against my abdomen. It has come to life from when I stroked it, and it is so hard and thick. I continue to kiss you and my lips move down your neck and behind your ear. I nibble the secret spot right behind the lobe and then nip the lobe as well.

You slide me down on your cock and move us into the stream of warm water. Water cascades over our bodies. It creates friction as we move together. You push me against the wall as the water pounds into our skin. I am bouncing on your cock. It is so hard, and fills me perfectly. You manage to reach to my clit and rub it,

Continued …

your hand moving between our bodies. I am gasping in pleasure and begging for more. You fuck me hard against the bathroom wall and it seems like only a few minutes, before we both cum together in unison.

I scream that I am cumming and my walls grip you so tight they milk your cum from you. I feel you shooting up my hole, and we explode in orgasmic pleasure. You lower me onto my shaky legs. We wash each other before finally leaving the shower, but not before, we play some more.

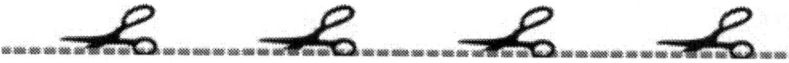

Prostitute

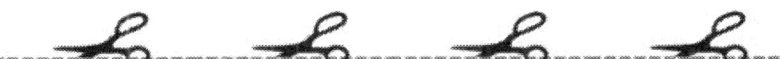

Tonight's The Night I have sex with a prostitute. I have always wanted to fuck a prostitute -- tonight you are my prostitute.

We arrange for me to pick you up somewhere. I want you to wear something slutty. We should meet in a bar or restaurant.

I drive you to a nearby hotel where I have booked a room for the night. I invite you in. You tell me how much it costs for a blowjob, and I tell you I want the whole shabang. You laugh and act coy and tell me that it is going to cost $500. I laugh and try to negotiate for a lower price, but you do not budge.

Finally, I agree. I set five crisp $100 bills on the table and tell you it is yours after you fuck me. I then let you take over. You remove my pants. You fondle my balls, and tell me how big my cock is. You get on your knees and suck it like the whore you are, and I grip your head holding you as I thrust my shaft deep into your throat. You suck it until I pull you off, and then I stand and move to the bed.

Once I get to the bed, you put the condom on my dick.

Continued ...

You then jump on top of it. You ride my cock, and I degrade you by calling you a whore, a slut, worthless, and a variety of other things. You are my prostitute for now so I can humiliate you in such a way.

You ride me until I cum shooting into the condom. You do not get to cum though. Most prostitutes only pretend to cum anyhow. Once I have cum you remove the condom and suck the cum off my dick. You clean me as I lie on the bed. I cover myself up and you fix your slut clothes.

You take the money and put it in your bra, hiding it away. You then leave the hotel room, and return to your car on your own as I bask in the memory of my prostitute experience.

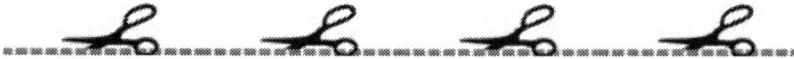

Mmmmm ... Latex

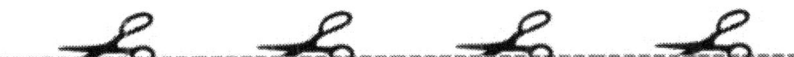

Tonight's The Night you dress in latex and wield a crop.

I can't believe how amazingly hot you look as the latex molds to your body. Your breasts jut out against the confining material and I lick my lips in anticipation.

"Darling -- you look beautiful in latex."

Without further warning, you grab the hair on my head.

"You want it sweetness don't you!" you shout.

I manage to pant out a "yes" before you drag me onto the floor.

You smack me on the ass with the crop and I blink. You instruct me to get undressed. You are dangerous with that thing. I get undressed, and my cock is semi-hard. It must be that delicious latex you are wearing.

Again, your strike makes me jump. You instruct me to get on my knees. I do. You are wearing black high heels that go together well with the black latex pants. I feel the stirring in my cock as it grows. You have me lie on my back though I do not know why.
Continued ...

"Now look at this, a big tough guy like you laying here naked in front of a nice little girl like me," you taunt, "what shall I do with you?"

You lean down and smack my cock with the crop. You then press the tip of the high heel into my balls. I scream. It hurts like a bitch, but you just laugh. You walk on my chest, and leave heel indentations on my skin. By now, I am almost crying.

"I want to see my boots worshipped properly. Do you know what I mean? I want them kissed and licked and I want you hard. Don't disappoint me."

You make fun of me, calling me a sissy. I guess I am. You spank me with the crop and then put your heel to my lips. You tell me to suck it and without hesitation, I do. You are my Goddess now and I worship you. You tell me to kiss up your foot. I do. I lick along the top and up your latex clad leg. The latex is driving me wild. I cannot believe how torturous you are by wearing it.

You lean over so your breasts are in my face. You allow me to lick your latex. I lick against the nipples and you lower the crop down to my cock again. You start beating me with the crop, telling me I am worthless. You tell me I am nothing. I can only nod as each stroke hits my balls and my cock.

You command me to worship your latex. I lick over it, over your body on your tits, your stomach and lower, against your well-defined snatch. I lick between the

Continued …

indent in the latex where your lips are. I lick the spot I believe is your clit and you rock against my face. I worship every inch of you as you continue to beat me with the crop.

"I know I don't deserve your love and I accept any punishment necessary to correct my bad behavior but I beg you ... play with my cock. Use me for your amusement. Take pleasure in knowing I am yours and yours alone," I beg.

Frowning at me, you reply, "Not tonight!"

Hand Job While Driving

Tonight's The Night that we take a trip.

Let's get away from the hustle and bustle of our daily lives. Pack up the car; we are leaving for the weekend. We can spend our time making love all-day and fucking in various places all night.

"Sure Honey, let's go."

We head off to a beach resort a few hours drive from where we live. It is dark when we start out.

There are very few cars on the highway. Our SUV seems quite lonely as it drives amidst only the few lone trucks that are out all night. I have a secret plan that will make you happy.

We've been driving for about 15 minutes when I slide over closer to you. You smile and I rest my head on your shoulder. I then slide my hand down to your crotch. Your eyes widen, but you know that I have an adventurous streak so you let me fondle you through your jeans.

I unzip them and you ask me what I am doing. I don't reply, save for my devilish grin. Once your jeans are open, I reach in your boxers and pull out your cock.

Continued …

You have a huge smile on your face, but you try to focus on driving. I can see that you want to close your eyes and enjoy the feeling, but you know you can't. I unbutton your shirt.

I flick my tongue and suck your nipples while rubbing your now massive cock. I lean down long enough to swipe the head of your penis with my tongue and give it a soft kiss. I wrap my hand around the shaft and slowly I stroke. I stroke up and down the whole length of you.

You begin to groan in pleasure but your eyes stay focused on the road. My hands are rubbing your balls, rolling them around in my palm.

I move back up and take the shaft into my hand again. I stroke softly and then faster. I build up momentum and as I do, I build up the pressure on your cock. You swerve a little but correct the SUV easily. I am stroking faster now, rubbing up and down like wild. I am gripping you in my palm tightly and you are fucking my hand, thrusting your hips. You fight to keep the car under control.

I can feel your cock twitching. I can feel the stirrings and I start talking dirty to you. I tell you I'm your whore. I tell you all the dirty things I am going to do to you while we are on vacation. All you can do is grind your hips and when you are ready to cum I lean down and let you shoot into my mouth.

Continued …

"Oh, my effin' god!" You cry as you detonate.

I lick the cum off you, while still rubbing your cock and balls. I suck up every drop, and you don't even stop the car. I lick my lips and sit up. I give you a seductive wink to tell you there is much more to come.

"Well, I guess you did start this trip right." you say.

"It's not over yet," I say, "Now let's get there and do it again!"

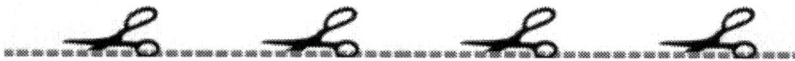

Double Dong

Tonight's The Night we play with a double dong.

"Are you ready to give up that virgin ass of yours?" I ask you.

You just grin. You take off your clothing as I take off my robe.

"Turn around and get on your hands and knees," I command as I lube up your tight, virgin ass and run the dong along your hole. "After tonight you'll understand how sexy your ass is to me."

I cup your balls in one hand, squeezing them slightly as I lean over and slide the toy between your cheeks. You moan and groan as the dildo teases you and soon you are pushing back against it. You gasp as you feel it but I slowly push it inside you. Your hips thrusting faster onto the dildo and you screech louder as you can feel the sensations run all the way up to the head of your cock.

Once the dildo is inside you, I spread my legs and slide the other half inside me. I hold the middle and feed it back and forth so we fuck it at the same time. The dildo slides in and out of us both, your ass and my pussy. Continued …

You scream loudly and thrust back against the invasive toy, I lean over and grab your cock as I fuck myself with the dildo and begin stroking your cock.

"How badly do you want this ass to be fucked? How badly do you want to feel it filled?" I ask, while thrusting the dildo in and out repeatedly.

I purr dirty words in your ear as I fuck us both and stroke your hard dick. I clench your cock harder and stroke faster as the excitement builds. We are both clenching around the dildo.

Your screams become louder, more persistent, as your body is ready to blast off. I place my head between your legs and begin licking the head of your engorged cock. I feel it twitch as I slowly, gently suck the head letting you cum on my waiting tongue. My hands caress your ass cheeks as you cum.

I pump you until there is nothing left and slowly slide the dildo from your ass and from my cunt. You are spent.

"I promise we will play again soon," I whisper.

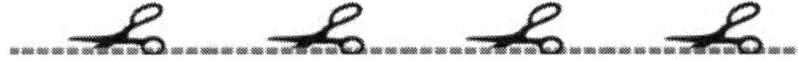

Be My Stranger

Tonight's The Night we play out a fantasy about someone finding me in a bar and fucking me on the dance floor.

We are at a club. I'm at the bar, when you ask me to dance. I agree. The beat and the movement of our hips and our bodies against each other are perfect. We dance for one song and then you move me back into the darker area of the dance floor, near the wall.

You press me against the wall and kiss me. I push you away but your persistent tongue leaves me begging for more. You pull me closer and rub your hands on my ass. You continue to rock against me as if we were dancing and I would breathe into your ear as I could feel your cock through your pants.

"What the Hell, we only live once. I want it tonight; I want something I would always remember. Let's enjoy."

You press your cock against me and you whisper in my ear that you are going to fuck me. You unzip your pants but you're so close to me that no one notices. I'm not wearing any panties under my skirt and it's so dark that when you pull my legs apart no one even notices.

Continued …

Your cock slides up me while we are standing up and though it appears we are dancing there is much more going on. The music is pumping all around us and your cock is pounding like mad into my tight little hole. You lift me up and wrap my legs around you and no one even notices a thing.

Other people on the dance floor cannot hear my grunts because of the music and it just appears that we are over affectionate and maybe a little drunk. Still I ride your cock, bouncing on it as I hold on to your waist. I fuck you harder as you hold me up. I start blowing in your ear, nibbling on it, as you hold me still and pound into my hot pussy.

The friction and the tease of your dick forced into my tight hole are driving me crazy. You mutter into my ear that you are going to cum and tell me you want me to cum with you. You continue to hold me and in a series of long violent thrusts we cum together. We both are barking like dogs in heat, but the music drowns us out.

I slide down your body until my feet are on the floor and you hold me to you, until my legs regain their stance. "So," you say with your arms still around me, "When are we going to have an interesting experience? We could try it at the store! You know a standing fuck in the dressing room at Bloomingdales. Wouldn't that be cool? Do you want to try that?"

We laugh as we go to the bar and order some drinks.

Birthday Spankings

Tonight is my birthday and I know that you won't let me down. I saw the present, one semi-large box and nothing else.

I ask to open it but you tell me we must wait. You feed me dinner and make me eat slowly, even though I try to rush. You offer me a glass of wine, which I take. Then it is time for the birthday cake. I have a slice because it is my favorite, but I am bursting at the seams and want to open my present.

Finally, you tell me it is time. I pick it up and rip off the wrapping much like a child on Christmas. Puzzled, I stare at the gift. It is a rather large paddle. You see the puzzled look on my face and you smile. You tell me that I shouldn't worry.

"This isn't your real present. This is just for some fun," you inform me.

I still have a puzzled look on my face and you take my hand and stand me up. You tell me to place my hands on the table and I do as you ask me. I scream as the first smack of the paddle cracks over my ass. "Whoa … what the hell …" You tell me that is one and that I should keep track. There are 26 more to go.

Continued …

You smack my ass and slowly it becomes redder with each strike. I wince, recoil and eventually tears sting my eyes because the pain is overwhelming. You do not stop -- you just keep spanking. These are my birthday spankings you tell me. You cannot stop.

I breathe a sigh of relief as you get near 25 and then finally number 26, and it is over.

"Can you fuck me now?" I beg.

"Are you ready...."

"Ohmigod, yes!" I plead as I feel your cock shoved up my cunt. You fuck me and caress my red ass with your free hand as I cry out in bliss.

I gasp and whimper as you fuck me and I beg for release. This is all so new to me. You smile, proud that I asked and you tell me it's OK to cum and me being the good girl that I want to be, I do as you tell me and explode.

The best birthday ever!

A Night of Blue Balls

Tonight's the night that you tease me. The answer will be the same all night long. "No, I won't make you cum. You are to do as I say at all times."

You love these games so you agree.

You have me undress, and lay down on the bed You grab my already fluffed up penis and give it a few strokes. Teasingly you bend over, careful to let me see your nice firm breasts, you swirl my engorged cock with your tongue.

"Play with you cock to keep it hard until I return - remember no cumming," You say as you disappear out the bedroom door.

You leave me lying in bed all by myself, with a massive raging hard-on. I reach down and grab my cock, pre-cum leaked out of the head and onto my hand. I bring my hand to my mouth and quickly lick it off, so that you don't think that I came. I stroke myself.

About ten minutes later, "Where is she," I ask myself.

I continue to stroke my hard as steel cock, careful to not bring myself to the point of orgasm.

Continued …

"It feels so good," I utter to myself as I squeeze my fingers against my balls. I'm so hard, that I could beat myself with a hammer, and it would feel good. "Where the hell is she."

"Looks like you are having a little bit of a problem," you say walking back into the bedroom. "Can I help in any way? Would you like me to suck it?" You nod. "OK, I'll suck it, but remember no cumming today."

I close my eyes and I feel fingernails playing with my balls and then hot lips on my cock. I open my eyes to see what you were doing to my cock. Your hand going up and down the length of my shaft, then digging your finger tips into the base of my shaft and squeezing my balls. Forget gently, almost with the whole force of you fingers you are squeezing. My cock starts to throb while screaming for release; suddenly you stop.

Frowning and scolding me, you order, "No cumming."

I squeeze and lock down on my PC muscles to prevent ejaculation, but my hot creamy semen is screaming to get out. My throbbing hard dick is bouncing back and forth, as I squeeze harder to prevent cumming. A thick glob of white love juice oozes out of my cock and the throbbing subsides. You lean over and grab the creamy juice with your tongue. You bring you lips up to mine, and kiss me softly. With your head nestled in my neck, you snuggle up to me and whisper, "Good Night Honey."

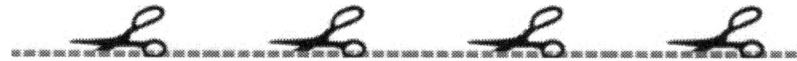

Edging with the G-gasm Method

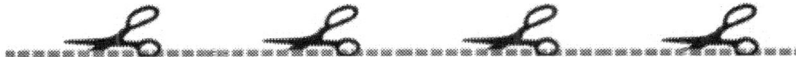

"Let me get your back," I say. I turn you around, take some soap from one of the wall-mounted canisters and lather you up. You close your eyes, tilt your head back and tell me how good it feels.

"That feels so nice," You say with my hands gliding over your slippery skin, glistening and wet. My erect penis slides up against your ass and settles between your cheeks – almost as if it was meant to be there.

You turn sideways to rinse off the soap. My hands continued to stroke you, one on your shoulder and breast the other moving down over your stomach and hips, the feelings tantalizing yet gentle. I slip my soapy hand into the crack of your ass and my other hand between your legs. I feel your pussy juices starting to flow, making you hot and wanting for more.

I slip a finger in your pussy with my thumb pressed against your clit --- you shiver unexpectedly. You arch your back slightly to get a better position against my fingers. You encourage me by stroking my throbbing cock vigorously. "Mmmmm," you whisper to spur me on. "This feels great."

Continued …

Standing at your side, my fingers have a perfect angle to reach your G-spot. Your G-spot is the size of a dime – you are ready. In your love hole, I gently insert a second finger. The fingers in your pussy plunge in and out setting a rhythm that has your hips moving, my thumb gently caressing your engorged clit.

My other hand is busy working the back door. I gently insert the tip of my finger inside your ass. You groan as the finger invades your other hole. You pushed back on it, wanting to feel your ass stretch around my finger.

"Oh fuck, so damn tight," You say as your ass deliciously squeezes my finger.

I reached to find your G-spot with my other hand. I start to stroke the now swollen love spot. You cry out with my fingers rubbing back and forth over your G-spot, my thumb massaging your clit, and around the other side of your body, a finger working your ass.

I hear the sloppy sound of my fingers in your wet pussy; it feels so good – so obscenely dirty.

"How do you like that - You hot cunt! You little slut! Is this good enough for you? You like these magic fingers in your tight little holes. That's my little whore! You are a slut, aren't you? You love it, don't you?" You love it when I talk dirty to you.

Continued …

"Oh hell yes!" you spit the words out from between your clenched teeth. "Yes I am a fuckin' slut! I am a whore; I'm whatever the fuck you want! Oh my gosh ... I am gonna ..."

I stop rubbing your G-spot as you approach climax. I pull my fingers from your pussy and bring them to my face, sniffing your juices before tasting them. You stick out your tongue and lick one of my goo covered fingers. You love the taste, and I sure liked what I am seeing – that really turns me on.

"Oh Baby give me some more ...," you whisper.

I reached back down to your love hole, it is slippery with cunt-juice and you sway slightly as I re-insert my fingers gently.

My other hand working your ass, I rub your soaking wet cunt a little rougher than before. A muffled moan burst from you when my finger stroked your aching love button. Spreading your legs, you move in rhythm with me as I draw slow and sensuous circles around your G-spot.

Your G-spot, swells to the size of a bottle cap as I rub it furiously. I feel you squeeze my finger with your pussy and ass, "Oh, fuck, baby that is so hot ... Oh, shit that's it ... I'm done, I'm gonna cum..."

Again, I pull my fingers out of your pussy; I want to prolong the first G-gasm as long as possible. I love teasing and playing by bringing you right up to the edge of G-gasm, and then stop rubbing for a few moments.

"Oh, god, that's good...," You let out, "More, keep doing it ... yes, give it to me ..."

"Yeah you dirty little bitch ...You like it in the ass --- don't you! Give me that pussy of yours bitch I want to make you squeal some more!" I continue.

My fingers found your G-spot again and I start to rub. Your pussy starts to shake and convulse. Waves of pleasure crash through your body, each G-gasm stronger than the last. Your wet walls squeeze my finger as it moved within you. I quicken the pace of me finger fucking your ass with one hand and rubbing your swollen G-spot with the other.

You explode into the wildest craziest G-gasm I have ever witnessed! It seemed to last forever! This G-gasm lasts for what seemed like several minutes!

Wrapping my arms around you, I pull you close, holding you tight. Your body convulsed so intensely I couldn't help but ask her if you are all right!

You whisper, "Ooooh my GOD ... that was fuckin' unbelievable ..."

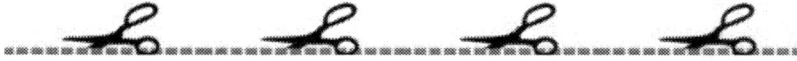

www.ingramcontent.com/pod-product-compliance
Lightning Source LLC
LaVergne TN
LVHW011425080426
835512LV00005B/273

Table of contents

Forward	7
Cock Worship	10
Night of Porn	13
No Cumming	15
One Free Flogging	17
Man in Panties	19
One Body Sundae	21
A Night of Bondage	23
Nibbles	26
Talk Dirty to Me	28
Sexy Dinner Date	31
Anal Evening	33
Master for a Night	36
Snowball	40
New Cock Jewelry	42
Exhibitionist	45
Little Slave Girl	47
Dr. Strangelove	50
Lap Dancing	52
Threesome	54
My First Anal Experience	56
Mutual Masturbation	58
Oily Massage	61
Let's Not Get Caught	64
That New Vibrator	66
Golden Shower	68
Working Girl	70
Ho! Ho! Ho!	72
I'm Horny	75
Voyeur Time	78
How Many Licks	80
Fisting	82
Wine and Dine Me	84
French Maid	86
A Sexy Cyber Fucking	88
My Porno Queen	91
Sex in the Shower	93
Prostitute	95
Mmmmm …. Latex	97
Hand Job While Driving	100
Double Dong	103
Be My Stranger	105
Birthday Spankings	107
A Night of Blue Balls	109
The G-gasm Method	111